Refreshing Infused Water Recipes

Simple, Healthy, and Hydrating Summer Beverages

BY

Alex K. Aton

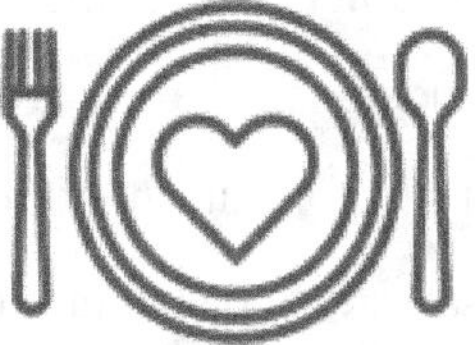

Licensing Information

It is strictly prohibited to engage in any commercial or non-commercial activity related to the content of this book without the explicit permission of the author. This includes, but is not limited to, selling, publishing, printing, copying, disseminating, or distributing the content in any form or medium. The author holds exclusive rights to the content and reserves the right to take legal action against any unauthorized usage.

If you have obtained an illegal copy of this book, please delete it immediately and obtain a legal version. Purchasing a legal version of this book supports the author's hard work and dedication in creating the content.

However, the author does not take responsibility for any actions taken by the reader based on the information provided in the book. The content is intended solely as an informational tool and the author has taken all necessary steps to ensure its accuracy. However, as with any information source, caution must be exercised when taking any steps based on the content of this book. It is advisable to seek professional guidance before taking any significant actions based on the information provided in this book.

Table of Contents

Introduction

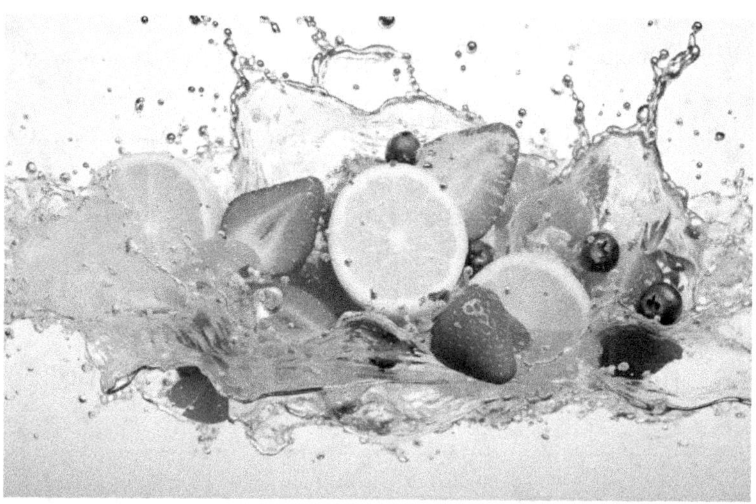

Are you tired of plain, boring water but want to stay hydrated throughout the day? Look no further! This book is your ultimate guide to making delicious and refreshing infused water recipes that will keep you sipping happily all summer long.

Inside these pages, you'll discover a wide array of easy-to-make drinks that combine the natural goodness of fruits, vegetables, and herbs with the simplicity of water. From classic combinations to unique and exciting flavors, there's something for everyone to enjoy.

Not only do these infused waters taste great, but they're also a healthy alternative to sugary beverages. By using fresh ingredients, you'll be able to take advantage of the vitamins, minerals, and antioxidants they provide, all while quenching your thirst.

Whether you're looking for a quick and easy way to liven up your daily water intake or want to impress guests at your next gathering, this book has you covered. With step-by-step instructions and helpful tips, you'll be able to create these delightful drinks in no time.

So, get ready to explore a world of refreshing possibilities and discover the joy of infused water. Your taste buds will thank you!

1. Classic Lemon Mint Cooler (aka Refreshing Citrus Splash)

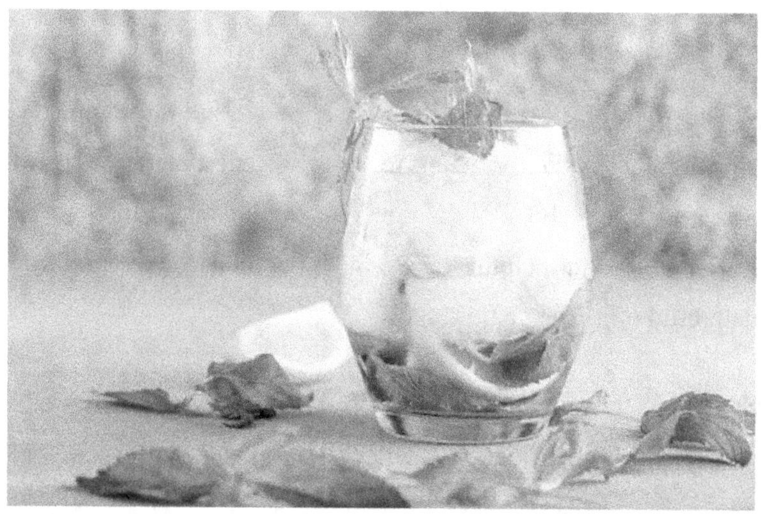

This classic lemon mint cooler, invented in the USA, is a popular summer drink that's easy to make. With just a few ingredients like fresh lemons, mint, and water, you can create a refreshing and thirst-quenching beverage that everyone will love. It's perfect for hot days and get-togethers with friends and family.

Preparation Time: 5 minutes

Cooking Time: 5 minutes

Serving Size: 4

Ingredients:

- 8 cups water
- 2 lemons, thinly sliced
- Juice of 1 lemon
- A few sprigs of fresh mint
- Ice

Instructions:

1. In a large pitcher, pour in 8 cups of cool water.
2. Squeeze the juice from 1 whole lemon directly into the water.
3. Thinly slice the remaining 2 lemons and add them to the pitcher as well.
4. Toss in a generous amount of ice cubes until the pitcher is almost full.
5. Pluck a few sprigs of fresh mint, give them a quick rinse, and place them in the pitcher.
6. Give everything a good stir to combine all the flavors.
7. Place the pitcher in the fridge for a bit to let the flavors mingle and the drink to chill.
8. Once the pitcher is nice and cold, pour the lemon mint cooler into glasses.
9. Serve to your thirsty friends and enjoy the refreshing taste together!

Special Notes:

- For an extra minty kick, try gently crushing the mint leaves before adding them to the pitcher. This releases more of that fresh mint flavor.
- Want to make it fancy? Freeze some lemon slices or mint leaves in ice cube trays and add them to the glasses when serving for a pretty presentation.

2. Refreshing Citrus Cucumber Water (a.k.a. Summer Sip Sensation)

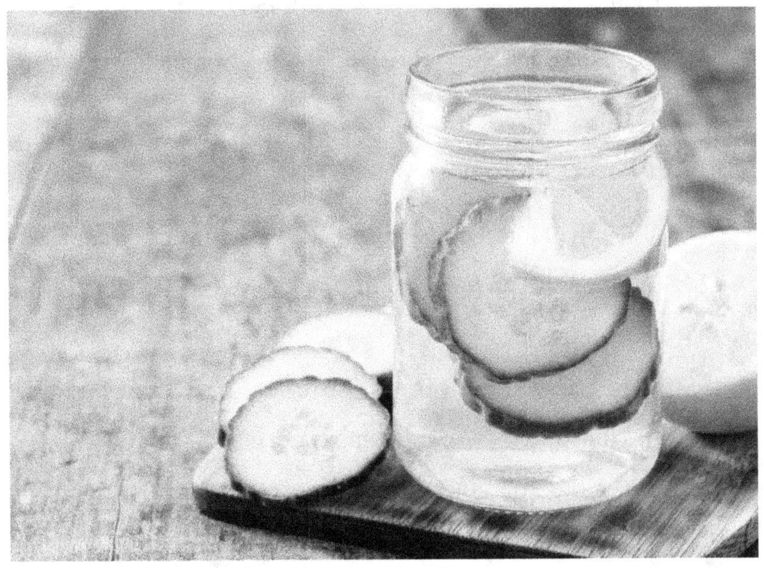

This thirst-quenching drink, inspired by the sunny beaches of California, is a hit at summer parties and picnics. With just a few simple ingredients like lemons, limes, and cucumbers, you can make a refreshing drink that everyone will enjoy. Perfect for staying cool on hot days!

Preparation Time: 5 minutes

Cooking Time: 5 minutes

Serving size: 4

Ingredients:

- 16 slices Cucumber
- 2 Limes (12 slices)
- 12 slices Lemon (about 1½ small to medium lemons)
- 4 cups Water

Instructions:

1. Slice the lemons, limes, and cucumber into thin rounds.
2. Grab a large pitcher, jar, or jug and toss in the sliced fruit and cucumber.
3. Pour the water over the citrus and cucumber slices, making sure they're fully submerged.
4. Cover the container with a lid or some plastic wrap to keep everything fresh.
5. Pop the mixture in the fridge and let it chill for 2-4 hours. This gives the flavors time to mingle and infuse the water.
6. When you're ready to serve, give the drink a good stir and pour it over ice in glasses.
7. Sit back, relax, and enjoy your refreshing Citrus Cucumber Water!

Special Notes:

- For an extra burst of flavor, try adding a sprig of fresh mint or a slice of ginger to the mix. It'll give your drink a tasty twist!
- If you like your drinks on the sweeter side, add a drizzle of honey or a splash of lemonade before serving. It's a sneaky way to satisfy your sweet tooth without going overboard.

3. Strawberry Basil Refresher (aka Summer's Secret Sip)

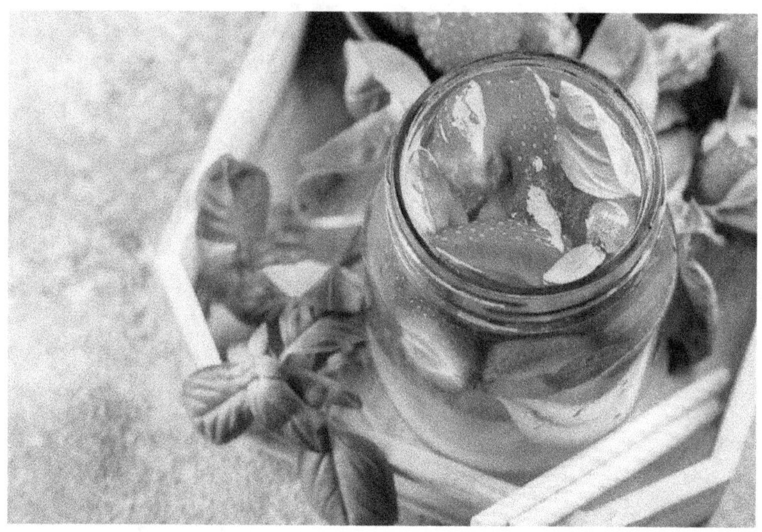

This thirst-quencher was born in sunny California and has become a hit at backyard barbecues across the country. With just a handful of strawberries, some fresh basil, and cold water, you can make a drink that'll have everyone asking for the recipe. Perfect for hot summer days!

Preparation Time: 5 mins

Cooking Time: 5 mins

Serving Size: 8

Ingredients:

- 8 cups cold filtered water
- 8-10 fresh basil leaves, lightly crushed
- 8 whole strawberries (fresh is best, but frozen works too)

Instructions:

1. Grab a pitcher and toss in the strawberries and crushed basil leaves.
2. If you're using fresh strawberries, use a muddler or the back of a wooden spoon to gently mash them, releasing their sweet juices.
3. Pour in the cold filtered water and give it a good stir.
4. Pop the pitcher in the fridge and let the flavors mingle for a few hours, or even better, overnight.
5. When you're ready to serve, pour the refreshing drink over ice and enjoy!

Special Notes:

- For an extra burst of flavor, add a slice of lemon or lime to each glass before serving.
- If you like your drinks on the sweeter side, stir in a touch of honey or agave nectar before chilling.

4. Raspberry Lemon Refresher (The Fruity Zinger)

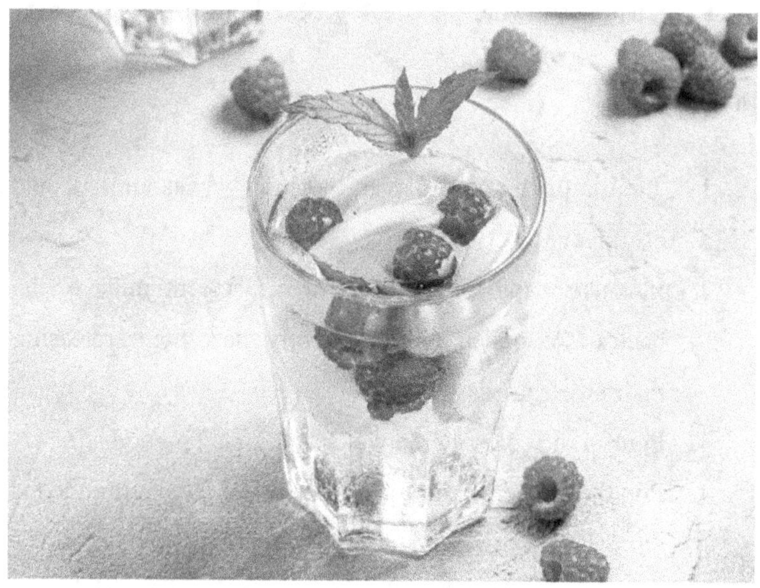

This refreshing drink, invented in California, has become a summertime favorite. With the tartness of lemon and the sweetness of raspberries, it's a perfect balance of flavors. You'll love how easy it is to make and how it quenches your thirst on hot days.

Preparation Time: 5 minutes

Cooking Time: 5 minutes

Serving Size: 8

Ingredients:

- 3 lemon slices
- 1 cup fresh raspberries
- 8 cups water

Instructions:

1. In a big pitcher or carafe made of glass, mix together the water, fresh raspberries, and lemon slices.
2. Put a lid on the container and stick it in the fridge for 12 to 24 hours.
3. When you're ready to serve, pour the mixture through a strainer to get rid of the fruit pieces.
4. Pour the strained drink into glasses and enjoy your refreshing Raspberry Lemon Refresher!

Special Notes:

- For an extra burst of flavor, muddle the raspberries and lemon slices a bit before adding the water. This releases more of their natural juices and makes the drink even tastier.
- Want to mix things up? Try adding a sprig of fresh mint to each glass before serving for a cool, invigorating twist.

5. Watermelon Rosemary Refresher (Minty Melon Quencher)

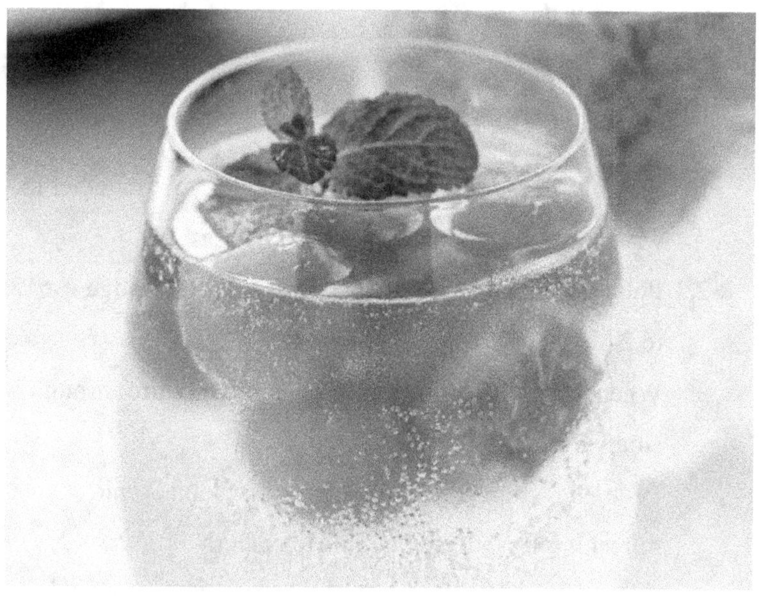

This refreshing drink was created in the southern US on hot summer days. It's become a popular way to cool off and hydrate with a hint of sweetness. The key ingredients are juicy watermelon and fragrant rosemary. Just a sip will make you feel revitalized.

Preparation Time: 5 mins

Cooking Time: 5 mins

Serving size: 8

Ingredients:

- 10 cups water
- 1 cup watermelon, cubed
- 2 stems fresh rosemary

Instructions:

1. Cut the watermelon flesh into small cubes and place in a large pitcher.
2. Gently crush the rosemary stems with your hands to release their aroma and add to the pitcher.
3. Pour in the water and stir everything together.
4. Place the pitcher in the fridge to chill overnight.
5. When ready to serve, give it a final stir. Pour into glasses over ice if desired.

Special Notes:

- For an extra minty zing, add a sprig of fresh mint to the pitcher before chilling.
- Turn it into a spritzer by topping each glass with a splash of sparkling water.

6. Orange Blueberry Infusion (Citrus Berry Blast)

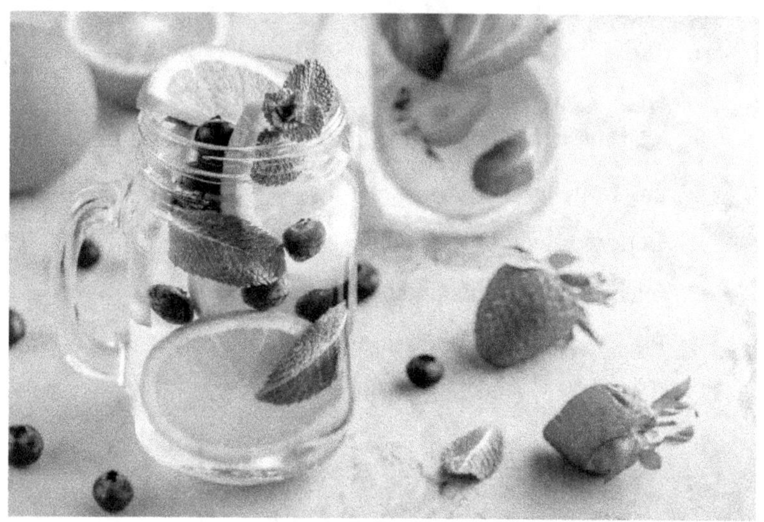

A fruity water infusion that started as a healthy hydration trend. Combining tart orange with sweet blueberries makes an irresistible flavor combo. Adding this to your daily water intake is an easy way to liven it up. You'll want to sip on it all day long.

Preparation Time: 5 mins

Cooking Time: 5 mins

Serving size: 8

Ingredients:

- 4 cups filtered water
- 1 orange, quartered
- 1/4 cup blueberries

Instructions:

1. Place the blueberries in a glass or bowl. Use the back of a spoon to gently mash them, releasing some of their juices.
2. Squeeze each orange quarter into a large pitcher, then drop the squeezed wedges into the pitcher as well.
3. Add the mashed blueberries and water to the pitcher. Mix well with a long spoon.
4. Chill the pitcher in the refrigerator for at least 2 hours, or overnight for more flavor.
5. Serve within 24 hours for best quality and taste. Pour into glasses, including some of the fruit.

Special Notes:

- Toss in a cinnamon stick while chilling for a hint of warm spice.
- Use sparkling water for a bubbly treat, almost like a natural soda!

7. Pineapple Mint Refresher (AKA Tropical Mojito Mocktail)

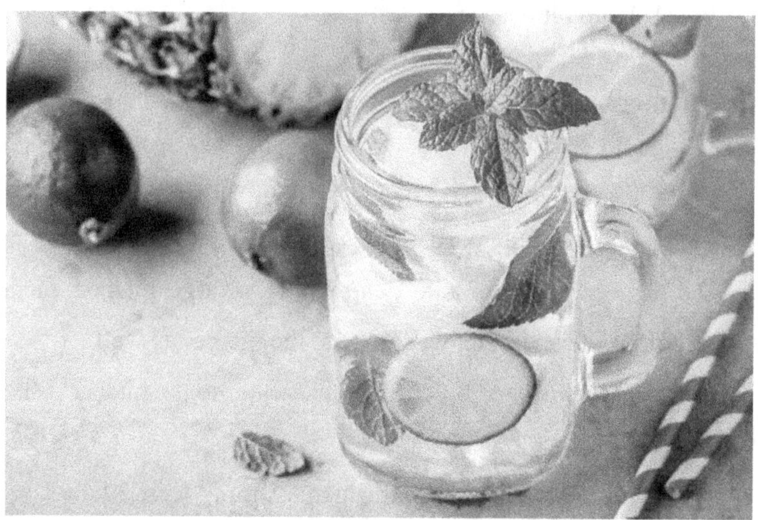

This thirst-quenching drink comes from the sunny beaches of Hawaii. It's a local favorite that combines the sweetness of pineapple with the cool freshness of mint. The main ingredients are just fresh pineapple, mint leaves, and water. You'll love sipping this on a hot day.

Preparation Time: 5 mins

Infusion Time: 12-24 hours

Serving size: 8

Ingredients:

- 3 fresh mint sprigs
- 2 quarts water
- 1/4 fresh pineapple, sliced

Instructions:

1. Get a big glass pitcher or carafe. Put all the ingredients inside it.
2. Put a cover on top and stick it in the fridge. Let it sit there for 12-24 hours so the flavors can meld.
3. When you're ready to drink it, pour it through a strainer first to catch the pineapple and mint.
4. Serve it up nice and cold. Enjoy!

Special Notes:

- For an extra minty kick, gently crush the mint leaves before adding them. This releases more mint oils.
- Toss in some ice cubes made from coconut water for a tropical twist.

8. Peach Ginger Splash (AKA Stone Fruit Spice Water)

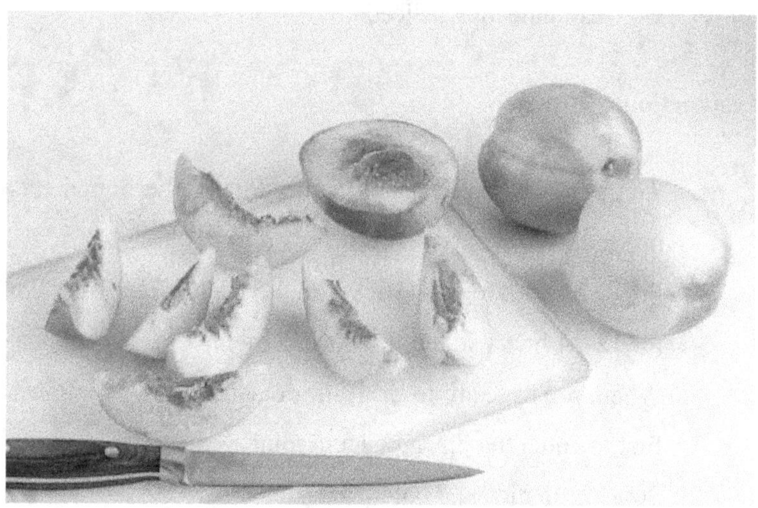

Born in the peach orchards of Georgia, this refreshing infused water is a regional staple. It marries the mellow sweetness of ripe peaches with the subtle heat of ginger root. With just 3 simple ingredients, it couldn't be easier to make. Perfect for porch sipping on lazy summer afternoons.

Preparation Time: 5 mins

Infusion Time: 2-3 hours

Serving size: 8

Ingredients:

- 8 ounces water
- 3 slices ginger, fresh
- 6 slices peach

Instructions:

1. Grab a mason jar and drop in the peach slices and ginger.
2. Pour the water on top until the jar is full.
3. Screw on the lid and pop it in the fridge for 2-3 hours to let the flavors infuse.
4. You can take out the peach and ginger before serving if you want, or leave them in.
5. Pour yourself a glass and enjoy!

Special Notes:

- For a prettier presentation, use a mix of yellow and white peaches.
- Freeze thin peach slices on a tray and use them in place of ice cubes so your water doesn't get diluted.

9. Cinnamon Apple Water (a.k.a. Apple Pie Hydration)

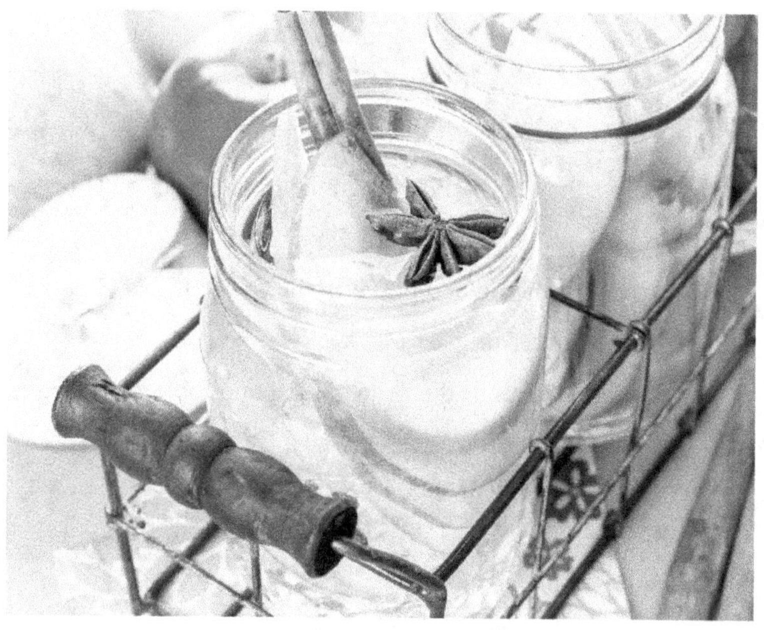

This refreshing drink was created by a health-conscious mom looking for a tasty way to stay hydrated. With just apples, cinnamon, and water, it's become a family favorite. The natural sweetness of the apples and warmth of the cinnamon make it feel like you're drinking a slice of apple pie. You'll love sipping on this throughout the day.

Preparation Time: 5 mins

Cooking Time: 5 mins

Serving Sizes: 1

Ingredients:

- 2 cinnamon sticks
- 1 pitcher of water
- 2 apples

Instructions:

1. Cut the apples into thin slices. No need to peel them.
2. Grab a pitcher and toss in the apple slices and cinnamon sticks.
3. Pour water into the pitcher until it's full.
4. Stick the pitcher in the fridge and let it chill for about an hour. This gives time for the apple and cinnamon flavors to infuse into the water.
5. Pour yourself a glass, and enjoy! Keep making this tasty water to stay hydrated all day long.

Special Notes:

- For an extra flavor boost, sprinkle a dash of ground cinnamon or nutmeg right into your glass before drinking.
- Try using different apple varieties to switch up the flavor profile. Honeycrisp will give a bolder sweetness while Granny Smith adds a nice tartness.

10. Rosemary Grapefruit Water (a.k.a. Citrus Herb Refresher)

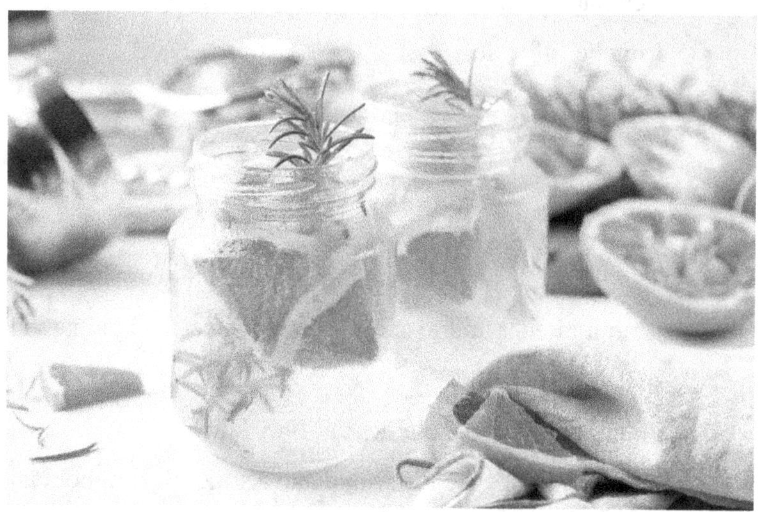

Invented by a yoga instructor, this water is loved by her students for its unique taste. The mix of tangy grapefruit and fragrant rosemary makes it a refreshing choice on hot days. With vitamin C and herbal benefits, it's a healthy way to quench your thirst. Even kids will want to drink more water with this delicious combo.

Preparation Time: 5 mins

Cooking Time: 5 mins

Serving Sizes: 4

Ingredients:

- 3 cups water
- 2 sprigs rosemary
- 1 organic pink grapefruit

Instructions:

1. Rinse off the grapefruit really well, especially if it's not organic.
2. Cut the grapefruit in half. Squeeze the juice from one half into a bowl. Slice up the other half and add the slices to the bowl too.
3. Toss the rosemary sprigs into the bowl with the grapefruit.
4. Pour in the water until the bowl is full.
5. Cover the bowl and let it hang out in the fridge for at least 4 hours, but overnight is even better.
6. When you're ready to drink, pour it into glasses. The rosemary grapefruit water is ready to enjoy!

Special Notes:

- Muddle the rosemary a bit with a wooden spoon before adding it to the water. This helps release even more of its aromatic oils.
- For a fancier presentation, add a slice of grapefruit and small sprig of rosemary to each glass before serving.

11. Cherry Limeade Water (a.k.a. Cherry Citrus Splash)

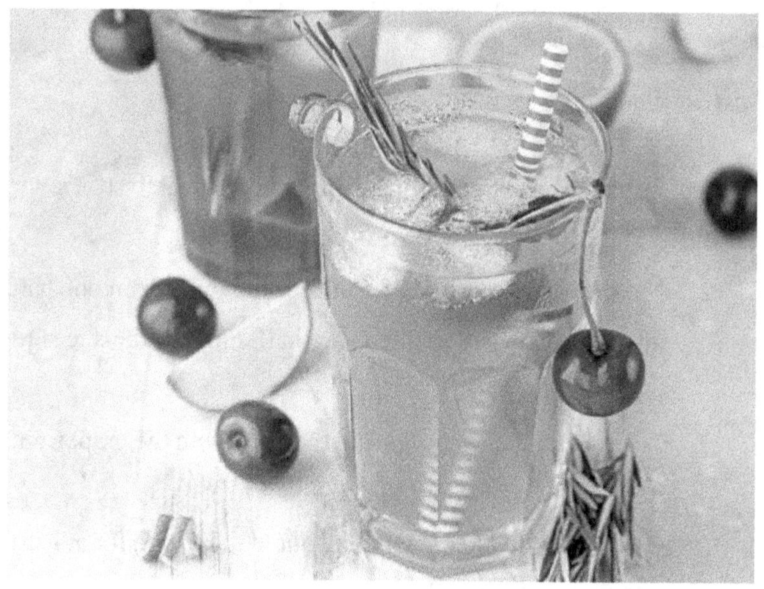

This drink was dreamed up by a mom who wanted her kids to drink more water. By adding cherries and lime to plain water, she created a healthier version of cherry limeade that the whole family loves. It's an easy way to keep everyone happy and hydrated, especially in the summer heat.

Preparation Time: 5 mins

Cooking Time: 5 mins

Serving Sizes: 1

Ingredients:

- 1 glass of water
- 2 lime slices
- 4 fresh cherries, pitted
- Ice

Instructions:

1. Fill a glass about 3/4 full with ice and water.
2. Drop in the lime slices and pitted cherries.
3. Give it a good stir.
4. Let it sit for about 5 minutes so the flavors can mingle.
5. Drink up, letting the cherries and lime hang out in the glass while you sip. It's like a cherry limeade but without any of the fake stuff.

Special Notes:

- For a fun grown-up twist, add a splash of tart cherry juice to bump up the cherry flavor even more.
- No fresh cherries? No problem! Thawed frozen cherries work well too.

12. Lemon Lavender Water (a.k.a. Floral Lemonade)

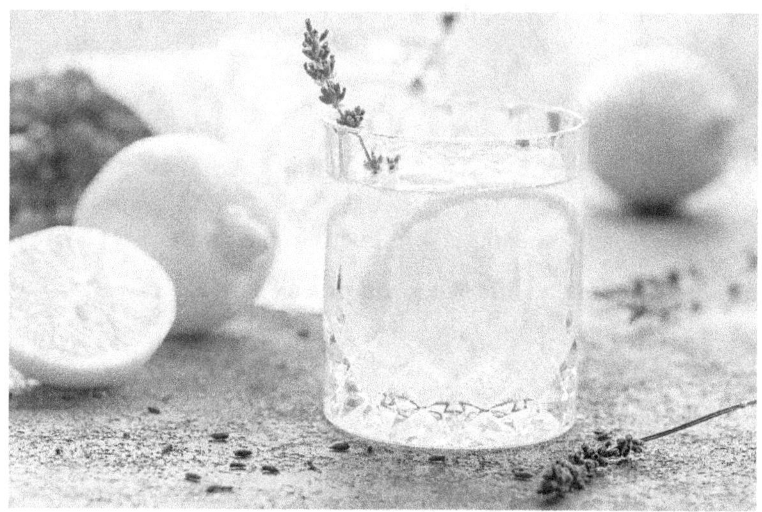

This elegant water was created by a tea lover looking to cut back on caffeine. The delicate floral notes from the lavender perfectly balance the bright lemon. It's become a hit at garden parties and baby showers. Sipping a cold glass feels like relaxing in the middle of a fragrant garden.

Preparation Time: 5 mins

Cooking Time: 5 mins

Serving Sizes: 2-4

Ingredients:

- 1 lemon
- 1 tbsp dried lavender buds
- 2 quarts cold water

Instructions:

1. Cut the lemon into thin slices. Toss the slices into a 2-quart pitcher.
2. Sprinkle the lavender buds over top of the lemon slices.
3. Pour the cold water into the pitcher until it's full.
4. Give everything a gentle stir to mix it up.
5. Pour into glasses and enjoy your lemon lavender water! Easy and so elegant.

Special Notes:

- Make sure to use culinary grade lavender buds, not stuff meant for potpourri or sachets.
- Crush the lavender buds a little in your hand before adding them to help release the oils and aroma.

13. Spicy Mango Water (Fiesta del Mango)

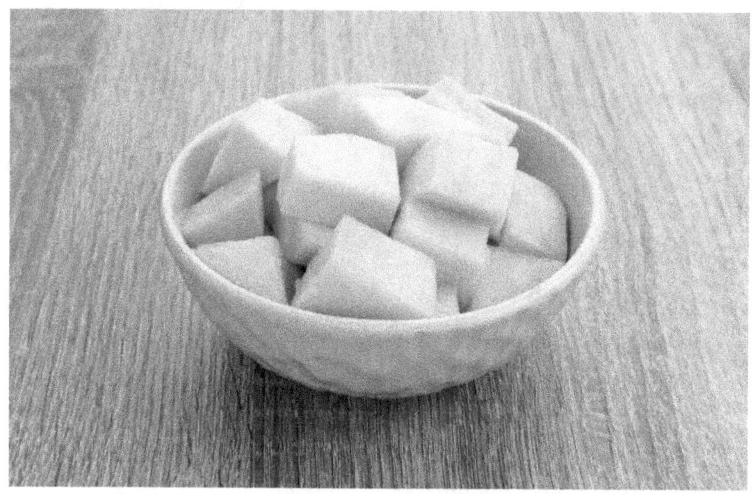

This refreshing drink comes from Mexico and is enjoyed on hot days. Mango and jalapeño are the key ingredients. You mix them with water and chill overnight. The result is a sweet and spicy flavor that'll wake up your taste buds. Perfect for sipping by the pool.

Preparation Time: 5 mins

Cooking Time: 5 mins

Serving Sizes: 8

Ingredients:

- 1/2 jalapeño, sliced with seeds removed
- 1 cup mango, chopped

Instructions:

1. Rinse the mango and jalapeño thoroughly.
2. Chop the mango into small pieces and slice the jalapeño, taking out the seeds.
3. Toss the mango and jalapeño into a 2-quart pitcher. Add cold water to the top.
4. Stick the pitcher in the fridge and let it chill overnight. This allows the flavors to really come out.
5. When you're ready to drink, give it a stir and pour over ice. The water stays good for 2 days in the fridge.
6. After finishing the water, eat the fruit pieces or blend them up into a tasty smoothie.

Special Notes:

- For an adult twist, add a shot of tequila or rum to each glass before pouring the mango water.
- Muddle the mango and jalapeño a bit in the pitcher to release even more of their flavors into the water.

14. Berry Sage Spritzer (Wisdom of the Woods)

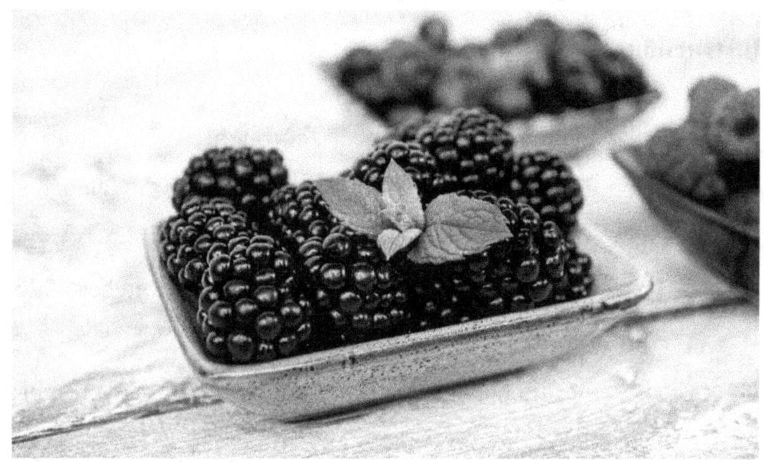

This berry and herb water is easy to make by the glass or pitcher. Blackberries provide a tart sweetness while sage leaves add an earthy freshness. Muddling helps the flavors mingle with the water. Serve it chilled for a wisdom-bestowing beverage straight from nature.

Preparation Time: 5 mins

Cooking Time: 5 mins

Serving Sizes: 4-6

Ingredients:

- 3 sprigs sage with the leaves attached
- 1/2 cup fresh blackberries
- Ice
- Water

Instructions:

1. Toss the blackberries and sage into a pitcher. Muddle them gently with a wooden spoon to release their essence.
2. Fill the pitcher about halfway with ice cubes.
3. Pour cool water over the ice to the top of the pitcher.
4. Chill the pitcher in the fridge until you're ready to pour and sip.
5. To make an individual serving, muddle about 5 blackberries and a few sage leaves in a glass, then add ice and water.

Special Notes:

- Swap the sage for mint, basil, or thyme to customize the herby flavor.
- Spike it with gin or vodka and a splash of tonic for a boozy berry cocktail.

15. Tangy Kiwi Cooler (Tropical Tonic)

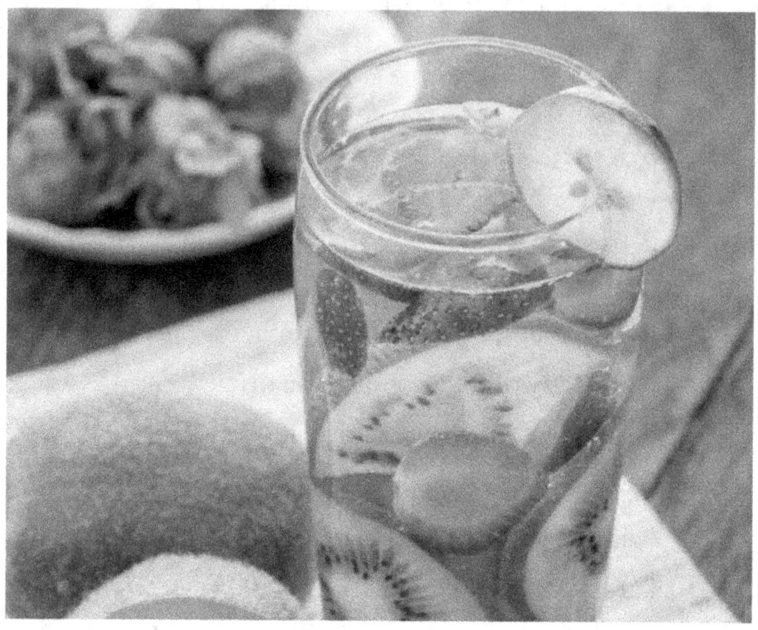

This fruity infused water comes from Europe and is a delicious way to stay hydrated. Kiwi, strawberries, lemon and herbs are the main stars. You just mix it all in a pitcher with water and ice. After chilling, you get a tangy, sweet drink full of vitamin C.

Preparation Time: 5 mins

Cooking Time: 5 mins

Serving Sizes: 4-6

Ingredients:

- 4-5 basil leaves
- 4 cups water
- 6-7 ice cubes
- 1 kiwi
- 1 lemon
- 5 oz strawberries
- 2 cardamom pods

Instructions:

1. Rinse the strawberries and remove the leafy tops. Slice them in half, then slice each half.
2. Peel the kiwi and cut it into thin rounds.
3. Cut the lemon into slices, leaving the peel on.
4. Pour the water into a pitcher. Add in the sliced fruit, basil leaves, and cardamom pods.
5. Plop in the ice cubes and place the pitcher in the refrigerator for at least 30 minutes before enjoying.

Special Notes:

- For a fizzy version, use sparkling water instead of still.
- Change up the flavors by trying different fruit and herb combos, like raspberry-mint or peach-thyme.

16. Pear Vanilla Quencher (Velvet Vanille)

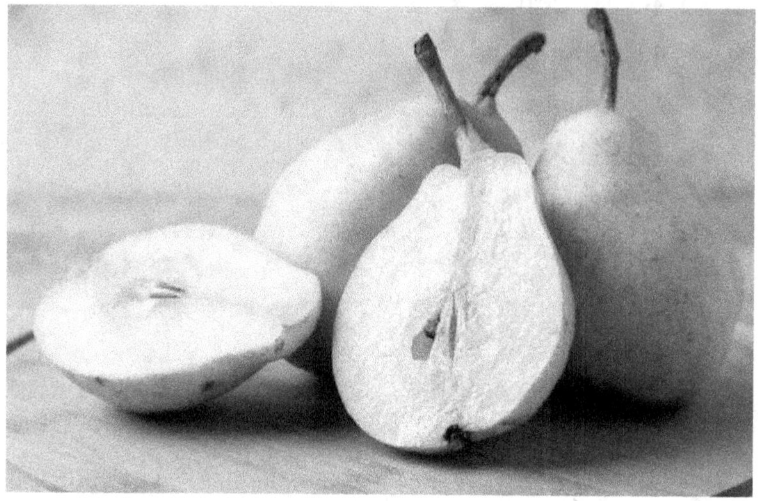

This infused water is popular in France for its smooth, sweet taste. Sliced pears and a whole vanilla bean lend a soft yet rich flavor to every sip. It only takes a few minutes to mix up a big batch that's fancy enough for a dinner party.

Preparation Time: 5 mins

Cooking Time: 5 mins

Serving Sizes: 2-4

Ingredients:

- 8 cups water
- 1 vanilla bean
- 1 pear, sliced
- Splash of vanilla extract

Instructions:

1. Slice the pear thinly, leaving the peel on for added nutrients.
2. Split the vanilla bean lengthwise with a sharp knife. Use the blade to scrape out the tiny black seeds inside.
3. Add the pear slices, split vanilla bean, and vanilla bean seeds to a large pitcher.
4. Pour in the water and add a small splash of vanilla extract.
5. Stir gently to combine. Chill the pitcher in the fridge for at least 30 minutes to allow the flavors to infuse.

Special Notes:

- Make it a cocktail by adding white wine or champagne in place of some of the water.
- Peel and core the pear before slicing for a smoother texture to the water.

17. Melon Cucumber Cooler (Oasis Splash)

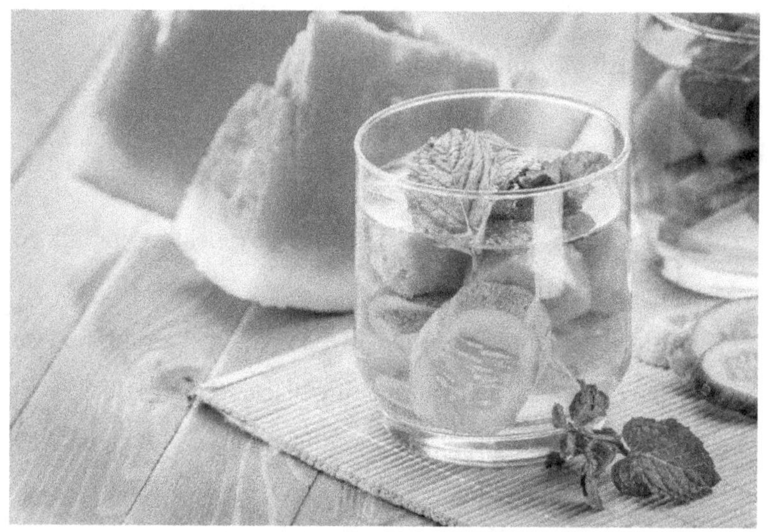

This spa water is like a mini vacation in a glass. Balled cantaloupe and thin cucumber slices float in icy water for a seriously refreshing drink. It's a breeze to stir together and only gets better as it chills. Hydration never tasted so good.

Preparation Time: 5 mins

Cooking Time: 5 mins

Serving Sizes: 6

Ingredients:

- 1 cucumber, sliced thin
- 3 ice cubes
- 5 cups water
- 1/2 cantaloupe, shaped into melon balls

Instructions:

1. Use a melon baller to scoop the cantaloupe flesh into little spheres.
2. Wash the cucumber and slice it thinly, discarding the ends.
3. Plunk the melon balls and cucumber slices into a pitcher.
4. Drop in the ice cubes, then pour the water to the top of the pitcher.
5. Give it all a good stir, then serve. It tastes even better after hanging out in the fridge for a while.

Special Notes:

- Float some fresh mint or basil leaves in each glass for an extra pop of flavor.
- Freeze melon balls on a sheet tray and use them in place of ice cubes to avoid diluting the water.

18. Figgy Fusion (Mediterranean Elixir)

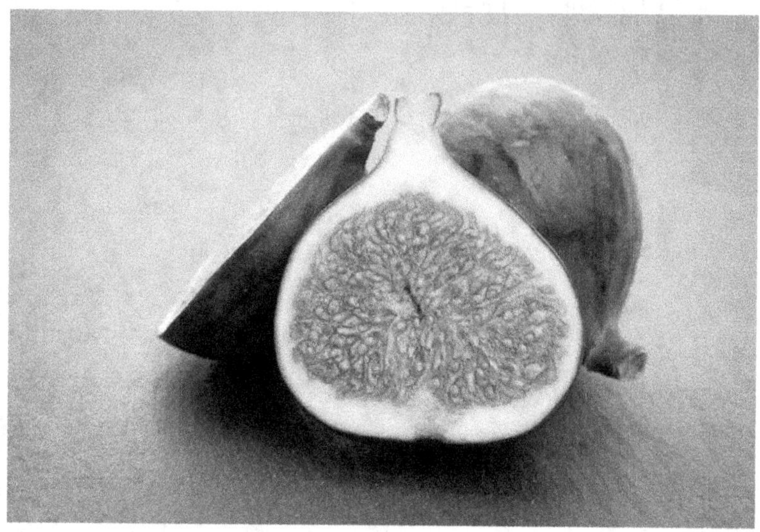

This infused water is a taste of pure sunshine. Fresh figs lend their honey-like sweetness to every swig. It's a cinch to make with an infuser bottle - just fill, shake and chill. After a few hours, you'll have a drink that would feel at home on the Italian coast.

Preparation Time: 5 mins

Cooking Time: 2 to 3 hours

Serving Sizes: 1

Ingredients:

- 15 fresh fig cubes

Instructions:

1. Chop the fresh figs into small cubes, about 1/2 inch in size.
2. Open the infuser bottle and place the fig cubes into the infusing tube. Twist on the tube's lid.
3. Fill the bottle about 3/4 full with water. The exact amount doesn't matter, just leave some room at the top.
4. Insert the tube into the bottle and tightly screw on the bottle's lid.
5. Give the bottle a few gentle shakes to distribute the figs.
6. Place the bottle in the fridge and let the water infuse for 2 to 3 hours before drinking.

Special Notes:

- Muddle the fig cubes a bit before putting them in the infuser to release more of their flavor.
- Add a cinnamon stick or star anise pod to the infuser for a warm spiced taste.

19. Plum Ginger Zinger (Spice Route Refresher)

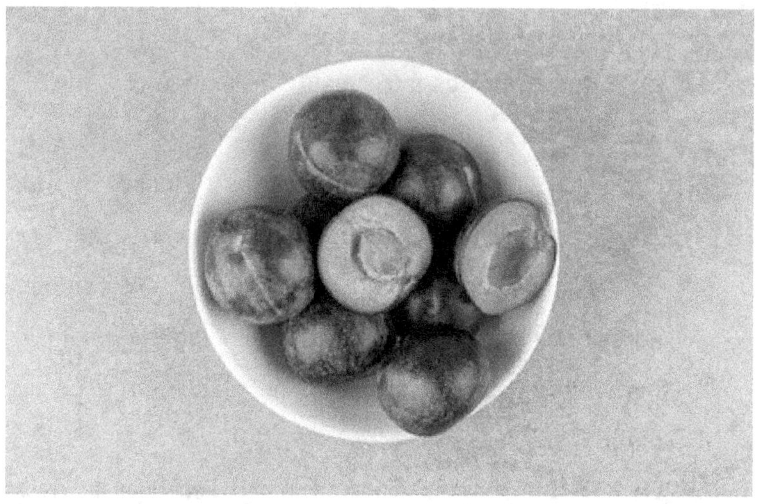

This infused water brings zing to a whole new level. Juicy plums and spicy ginger mingle for an eye-opening elixir. The flavors develop in a handy infuser bottle, so assembly is easy. A few hours of chilling later, and you're ready for an invigorating sip.

Preparation Time: 5 mins

Cooking Time: 2 to 3 hours

Serving Sizes: 1

Ingredients:

- 20 plum cubes
- 3 thick slices of ginger

Instructions:

1. Rinse and chop the plum into small cubes, roughly 1/2 inch each. You'll need 20 cubes total.
2. Peel the ginger and cut 3 thick coin-shaped slices, about 1/4 inch each.
3. Place 10 of the plum cubes into the infuser tube. Add the ginger slices, then top with the remaining 10 plum cubes. Close the infuser tube's lid.
4. Fill the bottle about 3/4 of the way with water. Drop in the infuser tube and tightly screw the cap onto the bottle.
5. Shake the bottle lightly to disperse the ingredients. Let it steep in the fridge for 2 to 3 hours to allow the flavors to infuse the water.

Special Notes:

- Freeze plum cubes and use them in place of ice to chill the water without diluting it.
- Steep some of the infused water with black tea for a zingy afternoon pick-me-up.

20. Strawberry Hibiscus Cooler (Red Nile Nectar)

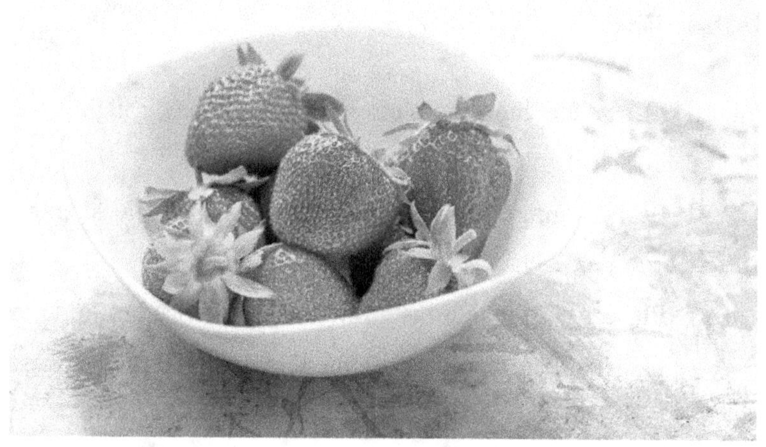

This ruby-hued water is like a drinkable gem. It combines dried hibiscus, strawberries and spices for a complex flavor. While it takes a bit of time to steep, the results are well worth it. Serve it over ice for a dazzling dose of hydration.

Preparation Time: 5 mins

Cooking Time: 30 mins

Serving Sizes: 4-8

Ingredients:

- 8 cups hot to boiling water
- 7-8 large strawberries, sliced
- 2 cinnamon sticks
- 1/2 cup dried hibiscus leaves
- 1 tbsp dried licorice root
- 1 tbsp dried ginger

Instructions:

1. Put a kettle on to boil 8 cups of water. While it heats up, prep the other ingredients.
2. Rinse and slice the strawberries, then add them to a large heatproof pitcher.
3. Measure out the hibiscus, licorice root, and ginger and add them to the pitcher, along with the cinnamon sticks.
4. Once the water boils, pour it into the pitcher over the other ingredients. Give it a stir.
5. Allow the mixture to steep for at least 30 minutes. The longer it steeps, the stronger the flavor will be. I recommend at least 2 hours.
6. When it reaches your desired strength, strain out the solids and pour the remaining liquid (about 6 cups) into glasses filled with ice.

Special Notes:

- For a more intense hue, steep for up to 12 hours in the fridge.
- Play with the flavor by adding other ingredients like peppermint leaves, lemongrass, or orange peel.

21. Papaya Lemon Infusion (Refreshing Tropical Quencher)

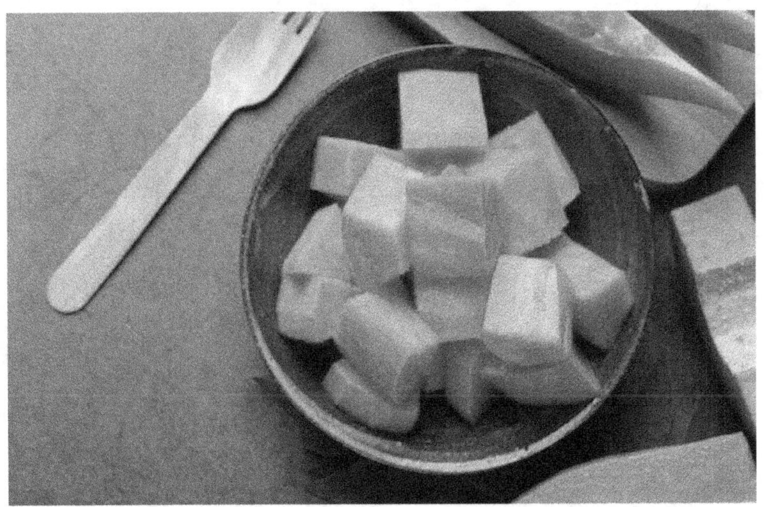

This thirst-quenching infused water originated in the tropics, combining the sweet flavor of ripe papaya with a zesty lemon twist. It's a popular choice for staying hydrated on hot summer days. The papaya and lemon infuse the water with a delightful taste that will make you crave more.

Preparation Time: 5 mins

Infusion Time: 2-3 hrs.

Serving Size: 1

Ingredients:

- 2 lemon slices
- 8 papaya cubes

Instructions:

1. Place 5 papaya cubes into an infusing tube, followed by the lemon slices and the remaining 3 papaya cubes. Close the lid of the tube.
2. Fill a bottle with water and insert the infusing tube. Tightly close the bottle's lid and give it a gentle shake.
3. Set the bottle aside and allow the water to infuse for 2-3 hours.
4. Once the lemony flavor has infused into the water, remove the lemon slices to prevent the water from becoming too sour or bitter.

Special Notes:

- For an extra refreshing twist, add a sprig of fresh mint to the infusing tube.
- Use chilled water for a more invigorating experience on hot days.

22. Apple Blueberry Burst (Fizzy Fruit Fiesta)

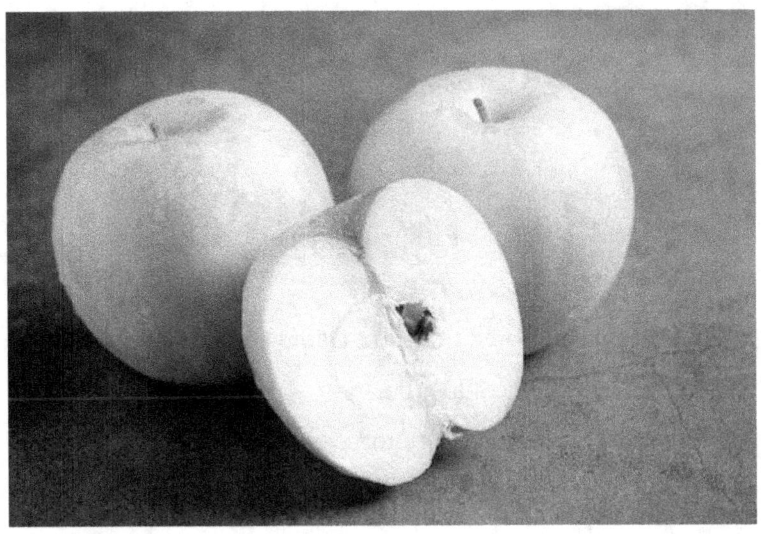

This effervescent blend of apple, orange, and blueberry is a hit at summer get-togethers. The combination of crisp green apple, juicy orange, and sweet blueberries creates a delightful fizzy drink that both kids and adults enjoy. It's easy to make and perfect for quenching your thirst.

Preparation Time: 5 mins

Cooking Time: 5 mins

Serving Sizes: 3

Ingredients:

- 1 green apple, preferred
- 1 cup blueberries
- 1 orange
- 24 fl oz cold water

Instructions:

1. Wash and chop the apple, orange, and blueberries into bite-sized pieces.
2. Add the prepared fruits to a Qarbo bottle and fill with cold water up to the 800 ml mark.
3. Carbonate the mixture to your desired level of fizziness using the Qarbo machine. Enjoy your refreshing drink!

Special Notes:

- For a sweeter drink, use a ripe, sweet variety of orange like navel oranges.
- Muddle the fruits slightly in the bottle before adding water for more intense flavors.

23. Raspberry Peach Spritzer (Sparkling Summer Sipper)

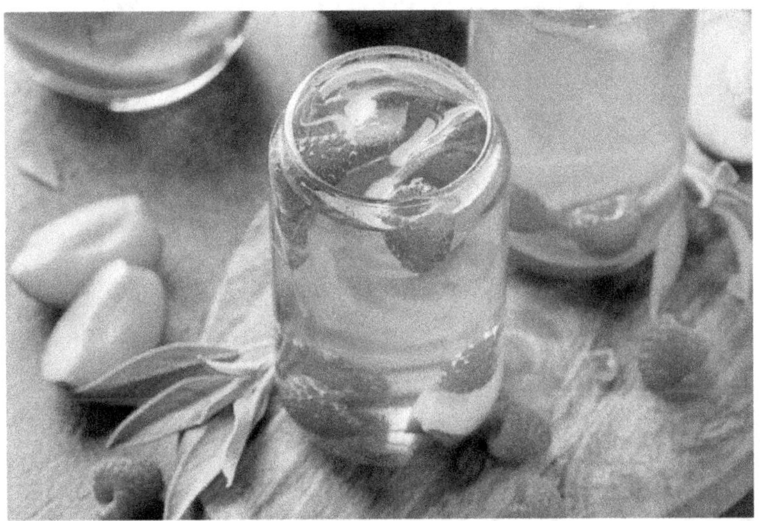

This effervescent raspberry peach drink with a hint of basil is a hit at barbecues and picnics. The combination of tart raspberries, juicy peaches, and fragrant basil creates a refreshing sparkling beverage that tastes like summer in a glass. It's quick to make and oh so delicious.

Preparation Time: 5 mins

Cooking Time: 5 mins

Serving Sizes: 1

Ingredients:

- 1/2 peach, sliced
- 3 basil leaves
- 1/2 cup raspberries

Instructions:

1. Add the raspberries, sliced peach, and basil leaves to your Spärkel bottle.
2. Fill the bottle with water up to the fill line.
3. Carbonate the mixture on level 3 using the Spärkel machine.
4. Pour into a glass, sit back, and enjoy your bubbly creation!

Special Notes:

- Gently crush the raspberries in the bottle for a more pronounced berry flavor.
- For a sweeter drink, add a dash of simple syrup or honey before carbonating.

24. Pineapple Coconut Refresher (Tropical Ginger Zinger)

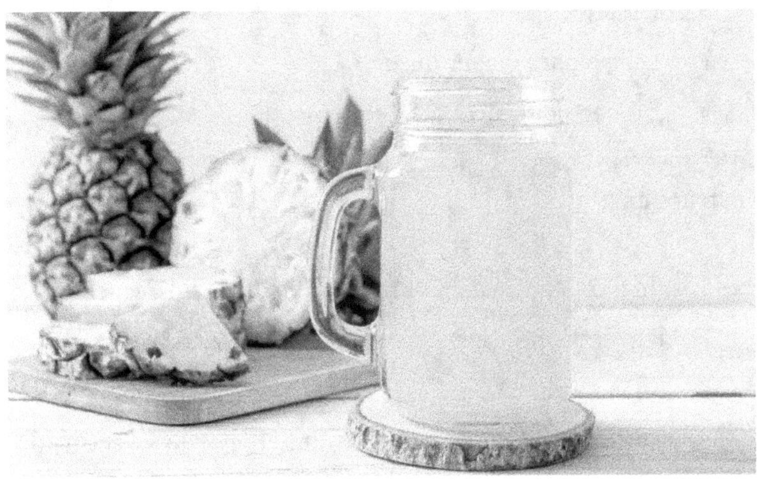

This invigorating pineapple coconut water with a kick of ginger is popular at tropical resorts and juice bars. The sweet pineapple pairs perfectly with hydrating coconut water, while ginger adds a subtle spicy zing. It's a tasty way to replenish electrolytes on sweltering days.

Preparation Time: 5 mins

Cooking Time: 5 mins

Serving Sizes: 2

Ingredients:

- 3/4 cup fresh pineapple juice
- 1 tsp honey, if needed
- 1 lime
- 1/2 tsp pure ginger juice
- 1/2 cup pure coconut water

Instructions:

1. In a cocktail shaker or mason jar filled with ice, combine the coconut water, pineapple juice, and ginger juice. Shake well.
2. Taste the mixture and add a little honey to sweeten it if needed. If your pineapple is ripe and sweet, additional honey may not be necessary.
3. Fill the glasses with plenty of ice cubes and thin slices of lime.
4. Next, pour the pineapple coconut water into the prepared glasses. If desired, finish with an extra squeeze of lime juice.

Special Notes:

- For a fun tropical twist, garnish with a slice of pineapple or a sprinkle of toasted coconut flakes.
- Make ice cubes from coconut water to avoid diluting the drink as the ice melts.

25. Cilantro Lime Cooler (Zesty Green Refresher)

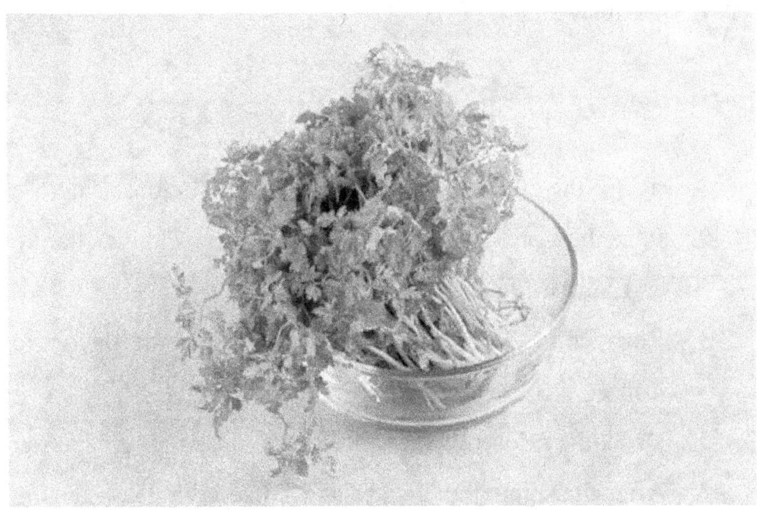

This invigorating infused water with cilantro and lime is beloved in Latin America. The fresh, citrusy flavors make it an ideal thirst quencher on hot days. Cilantro adds a unique refreshing taste that complements the tart limes perfectly. It's easy to make a big batch to sip on all day.

Preparation Time: 5 mins

Cooking Time: 5 mins

Serving Size: 8 cups

Ingredients:

- 1 1/2 cups fresh cilantro
- 2 limes, cut into thin wedges
- 7 cups water

Instructions:

1. Rinse the cilantro and limes thoroughly before using.
2. Pour the water into a large glass pitcher. Add the cilantro and lime wedges to the water.
3. Refrigerate the pitcher overnight to allow the flavors to infuse.
4. Drink the infused water within 24 hours for optimal taste. After that time, the cilantro and lime may release flavors that are too strong.

Special Notes:

- For a spicier version, add a few slices of jalapeño or a pinch of cayenne.
- Use sparkling water instead of still water for a bubbly, effervescent drink.

26. Grape Orange Splasher (Basil Berry Blast)

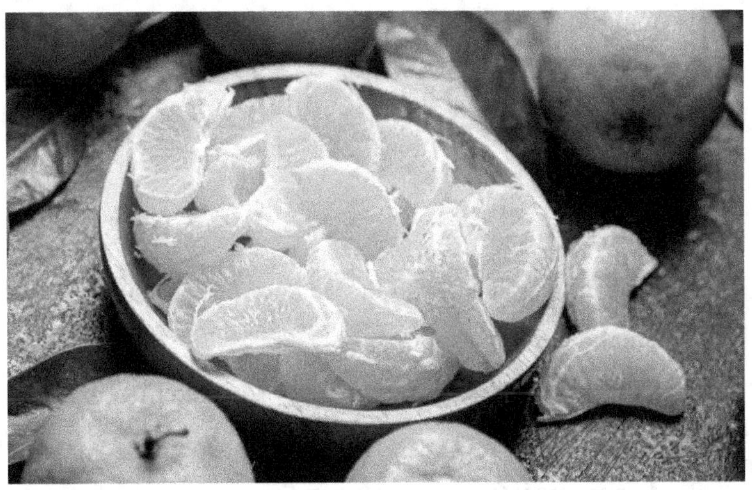

This refreshing blend of grapes, oranges, and basil is a crowd-pleaser at summer parties and picnics. The juicy fruits combine with fragrant basil for a delightful flavor that both kids and adults enjoy. It's a snap to whip up and tastes like sunshine in a glass.

Preparation Time: 5 mins

Cooking Time: 5 mins

Serving Sizes: 2

Ingredients:

- 1/2-gallon water or sparkling water
- 2 oranges, sliced (navel oranges preferred)
- 1/2 cup basil, chopped
- 1 cup red grapes, halved
- 2 cups ice

Instructions:

1. In a large pitcher, add the orange slices, chopped basil, and halved grapes.
2. Fill the pitcher with ice and then add water or sparkling water.
3. For a more intense flavor, cover the pitcher and refrigerate for at least 1 hour, or up to 2 days.
4. Pour into glasses, garnish with extra fruit and basil if desired, and serve chilled.

Special Notes:

- For a grown-up version, add a splash of gin or vodka to the pitcher before chilling.
- Freeze grapes and use them instead of ice cubes to avoid diluting the drink.

27. Pomegranate Lemon Infusion (Antioxidant Burst)

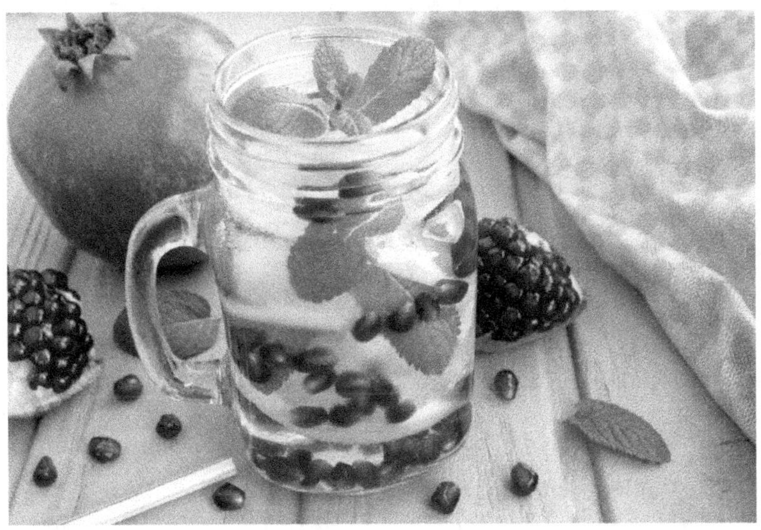

This refreshing infusion originated in the Middle East and has become a popular drink worldwide. The combination of pomegranate, lemon, and ginger creates a delightful flavor that's both tart and slightly spicy. It's a great way to stay hydrated while enjoying the health benefits of these powerhouse ingredients.

Preparation Time: 5 mins

Cooking Time: 5 mins

Serving Sizes: 8

Ingredients:

- 1 lemon
- 1 pomegranate
- 1-inch piece of ginger

Instructions:

1. Cut the pomegranate into sections and remove the arils. Put them in a large container and gently mash with a wooden spoon.
2. Peel the lemon, slice it, and add the slices to the container with the pomegranate.
3. Using a spoon, peel the ginger. Grate 1 tbsp of ginger and add it to the other ingredients.
4. Pour water over everything, then put the container in the fridge. Let it sit for 12-24 hours before serving.

Special Notes:

- For extra zing, add a pinch of cayenne pepper.
- Strain the infusion before serving for a smoother drink.

28. Nectarine Basil Clementine Cooler (Summer Sip Sensation)

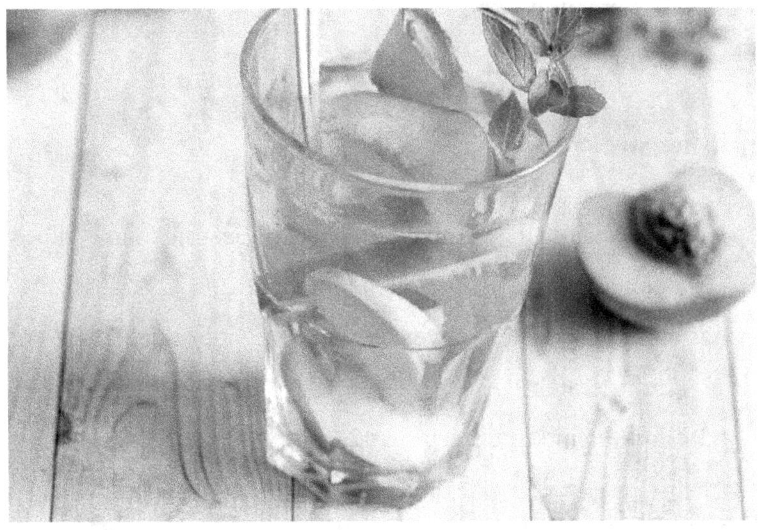

This delightful infusion is a taste of summer in a glass. It was created by a mixologist in California looking for a refreshing non-alcoholic drink. The sweetness of the nectarines and clementines is perfectly balanced by the herbal notes of basil. It's sure to become your new favorite summer beverage.

Preparation Time: 5 mins

Cooking Time: 5 mins

Serving Sizes: 6-8

Ingredients:

- 6 fresh basil leaves
- 1 medium nectarine, sliced
- 1 clementine, sliced
- 2 quarts water

Instructions:

1. Put the sliced nectarine, basil leaves, and sliced clementine in a large pitcher or carafe.
2. Add the water, cover the pitcher, and place it in the refrigerator.
3. Let the mixture steep for 12-24 hours for optimal flavor.

Special Notes:

- Use ripe, fragrant nectarines for the best taste.
- For a sparkling version, use carbonated water instead of still.

29. Orange Rosemary Refresher

(Herbal Hydrator)

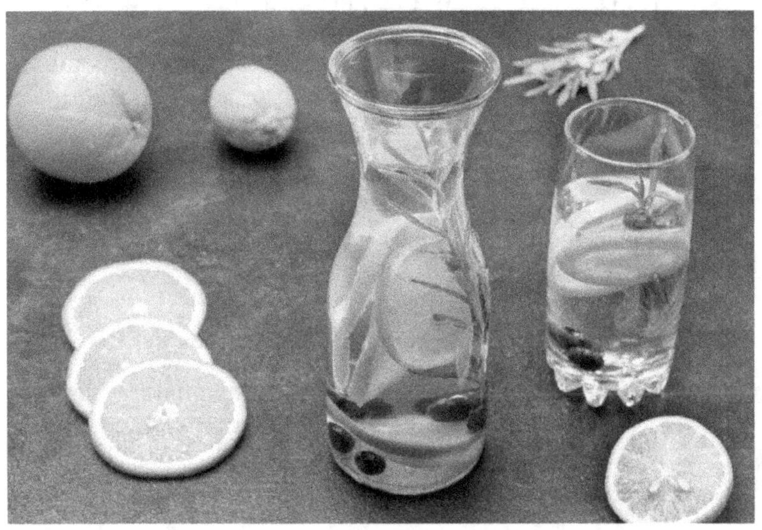

This invigorating infusion hails from the Mediterranean region, where both oranges and rosemary grow in abundance. The bright citrus notes of the orange are wonderfully complemented by the piney aroma of rosemary. It's a great way to stay hydrated and energized throughout the day.

Preparation Time: 15 mins

Cooking Time: 15 mins

Serving Sizes: 4

Ingredients:

- 4 sprigs rosemary
- 8-10 cups water (1.8-2.3 liters)
- 1/2 large orange, sliced and halved
- Additional orange slices and rosemary sprigs for garnish

Instructions:

1. Place the orange slices and rosemary sprigs in a large pitcher.
2. Pour the water over the ingredients in the pitcher.
3. Put the pitcher in the fridge and let the mixture steep for at least several hours, or overnight for best results.
4. When serving, pour the infused water into glasses or mason jars. If desired, garnish each glass with an extra orange slice and rosemary sprig.

Special Notes:

- Gently muddle the rosemary before adding it to the pitcher to release more flavor.
- For a sweeter drink, add a touch of honey or agave nectar.

30. Blackberry Citrus Splash (Berry Burst Blend)

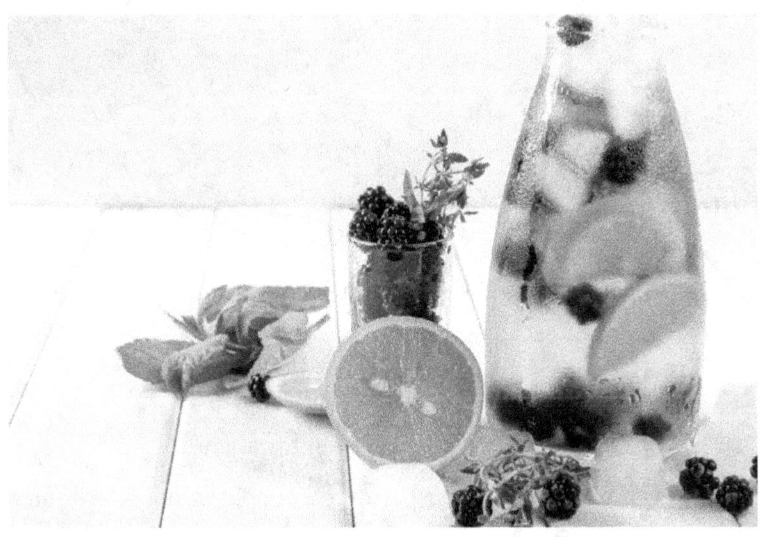

This refreshing infusion is a staple at summer barbecues in the American South. The combination of juicy blackberries and tart citrus is incredibly refreshing on a hot day. It's a healthier alternative to sugary sodas and a great way to use up summer berries.

Preparation Time: 5 mins

Cooking Time: 5 mins

Serving Sizes: 6

Ingredients:

- 1 lemon, sliced
- 6 cups water
- 1 orange, sliced
- 1/2 cup blackberries
- Ice

Instructions:

1. Put a few blackberries, orange slices, and lemon slices in a pitcher or carafe. Add ice.
2. Pour filtered water over the fruit and ice.
3. Place the pitcher in the refrigerator to chill.
4. The flavor will intensify after a couple of hours or more. Enjoy!

Special Notes:

- Mash the blackberries slightly before adding them to the pitcher for more flavor.
- For a fizzy version, top off each glass with a splash of sparkling water.

31. Watermelon Berry Blast (Summer Melon Medley)

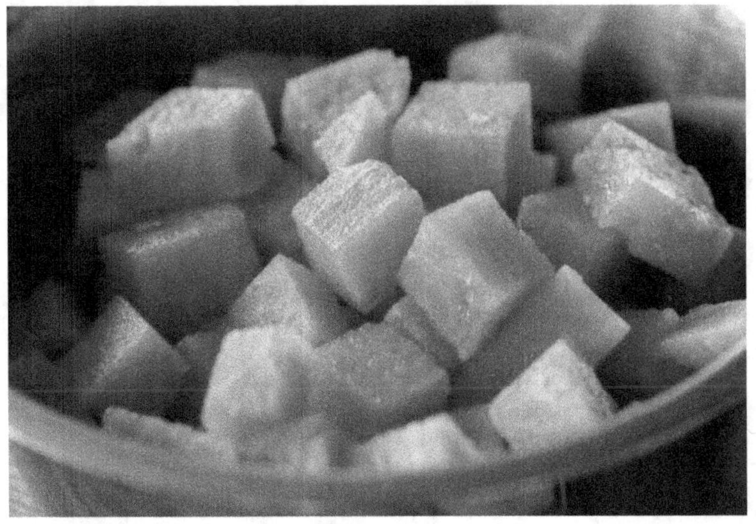

This delightful infusion is a hit at summer parties and picnics. It was created by a mom looking for a way to get her kids to drink more water. The sweet watermelon and tangy berries make it a refreshing treat that's loved by kids and adults alike.

Preparation Time: 5 mins

Cooking Time: 5 mins

Serving Sizes: 8

Ingredients:

- 1/2 cup raspberries
- 1/2 cup blueberries
- 1 gallon of water
- 1/2 cup watermelon, cut into pieces

Instructions:

1. Rinse the blueberries and raspberries. Add them to a pitcher that can hold a gallon or more of water.
2. Cut the watermelon into pieces and add it to the pitcher with the berries.
3. Pour 1 gallon of cold water into the pitcher.
4. Put the pitcher in the fridge for an hour to allow the fruit flavors to infuse into the water.

Special Notes:

- Use seedless watermelon for easier preparation and sipping.
- Freeze some of the fruit to use as ice cubes and keep your drink cool.

32. Kiwi Cucumber Cooler (Green Refresher)

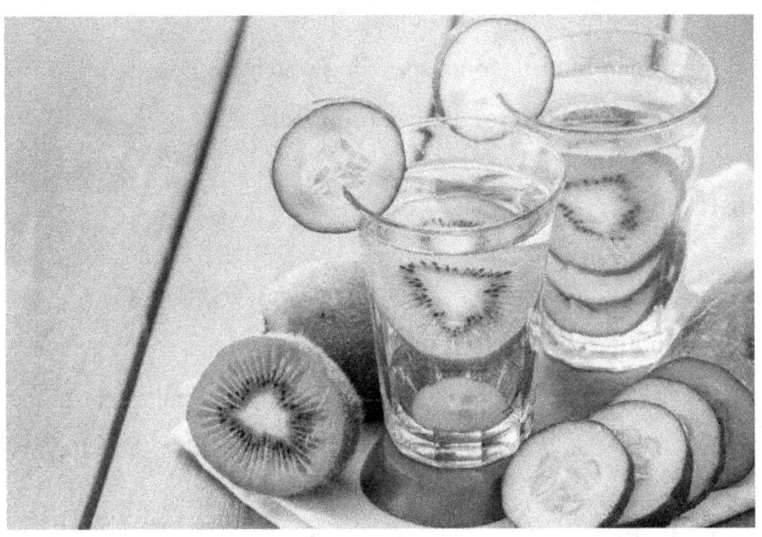

This unique infusion is a favorite among health enthusiasts. It was created by a yoga instructor who wanted a hydrating drink to serve after hot yoga classes. The mild sweetness of kiwi is balanced by the freshness of cucumber, making it a light and invigorating drink.

Preparation Time: 5 mins

Cooking Time: 5 mins

Serving Sizes: 1

Ingredients:

- 4 thin slices cucumber
- 2 thin slices of fresh lime, seeded
- 1/2 kiwi, peeled and thinly sliced
- 1 can lime-flavored sparkling water
- Mint or basil for garnish (optional)

Instructions:

1. Put the cucumber slices, kiwi slices, and lime slices in the bottom of a large drinking glass.
2. Using the back of a wooden spoon, gently mash the ingredients for about 20 seconds to release their flavors and juices.
3. Pour the lime-sparkling water over the fruit.
4. Add ice if desired and garnish with herbs.

Special Notes:

- Use a ripe but firm kiwi for the best texture and flavor.
- For a sweeter drink, add a teaspoon of honey.

33. Honeydew Cucumber Mint Infusion (Melon Mint Medley)

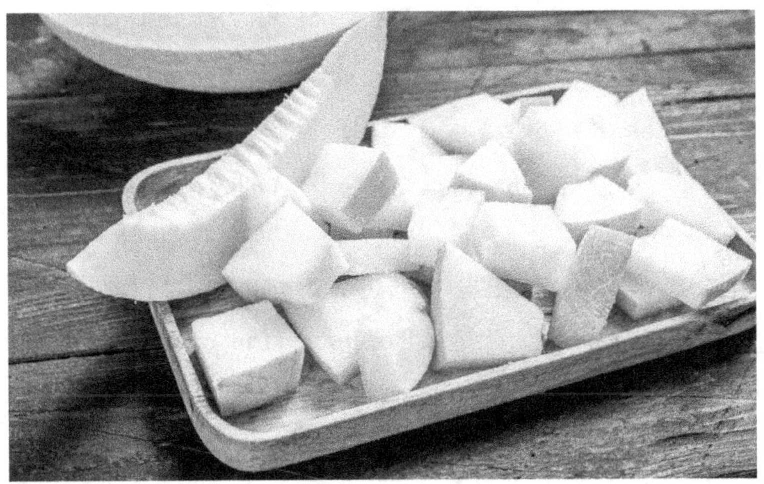

This refreshing infusion is a summer favorite in the southern United States. It was created by a bartender looking for a refreshing non-alcoholic option for patrons. The sweetness of honeydew, the freshness of cucumber, and the cool notes of mint make it an ideal drink for hot summer days.

Preparation Time: 5 mins

Cooking Time: 5 mins

Serving Sizes: 4

Ingredients:

- 1 cucumber, thinly sliced
- 1/2 cup honeydew cubes
- 10 fresh mint leaves, torn

Instructions:

1. Place the honeydew cubes, cucumber slices, and torn mint leaves in a large pitcher.
2. Add ice and fill the pitcher with water.
3. If desired, garnish with additional fruit or herbs.

Special Notes:

- For a more intense mint flavor, muddle the mint leaves before adding them to the pitcher.
- Try adding a slice of jalapeno for a spicy kick.

34. Pomegranate Pear Passion (Cinnamon Spiced Sip)

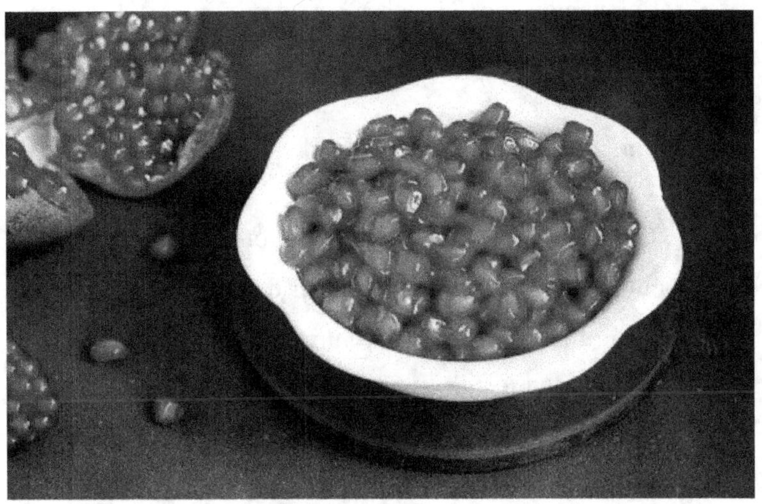

This warm and inviting infusion is perfect for cooler months. It was created by a barista looking for a unique alternative to hot apple cider. The tartness of the pomegranate is balanced by the sweetness of the pear, while the cinnamon adds a lovely warmth and spice.

Preparation Time: 5 mins

Cooking Time: 5 mins

Serving Sizes: 8

Ingredients:

- 1/2 small pear, sliced
- 1/4 cup pomegranate seeds
- 1 cinnamon stick (3 inches)
- 2 quarts water

Instructions:

1. Combine the water, sliced pear, pomegranate seeds, and cinnamon stick in a large pitcher or carafe.
2. Cover the pitcher and place it in the refrigerator.
3. Let the mixture steep for 12-24 hours.
4. Strain before serving.

Special Notes:

- For a hot version, heat the infusion in a saucepan before serving.
- Add a splash of pomegranate juice for a more intense flavor.

35. Lemon Ginger Turmeric Tonic (Golden Elixir)

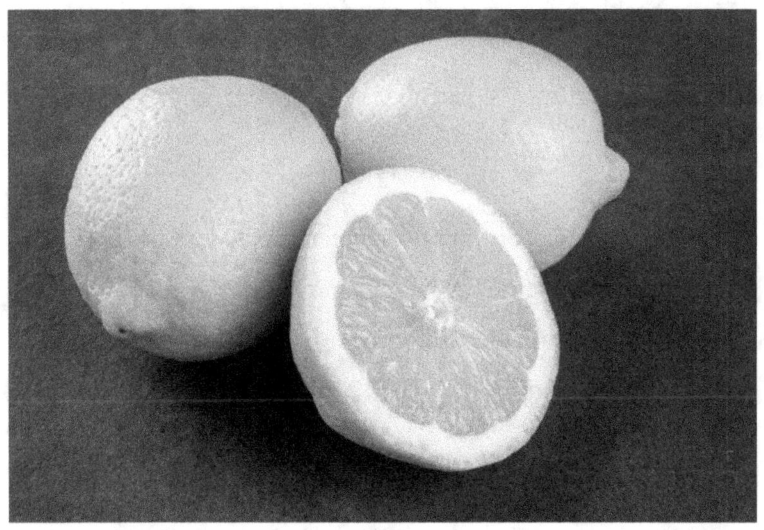

This vibrant infusion is popular among health-conscious individuals. It was created by a nutritionist looking for a way to incorporate the anti-inflammatory benefits of turmeric into a tasty drink. The zing of ginger and the tartness of lemon make it a refreshing and invigorating tonic.

Preparation Time: 5 mins

Cooking Time: 5 mins

Serving Sizes: 2 quarts

Ingredients:

- 4 slices fresh ginger root
- 1/2 lemon, sliced
- 1 tablespoon ground turmeric
- 2 quarts water

Instructions:

1. Combine the turmeric, ginger slices, lemon slices, and water in a large pitcher or carafe.
2. Cover the pitcher and place it in the refrigerator.
3. Let the mixture steep for 12-24 hours.

Special Notes:

- Add a pinch of black pepper to enhance the absorption of turmeric's benefits.
- Sweeten with honey or agave nectar if desired.

Conclusion

In conclusion, this book has been your guide to creating delicious and refreshing infused water recipes that make staying hydrated a pleasure. By exploring the various flavor combinations and experimenting with your own ideas, you've discovered just how easy and enjoyable it can be to liven up your daily water intake.

From the classic tastes of lemon and mint to the surprising and delightful pairings of watermelon and rosemary or pineapple and basil, you now have a wealth of options to choose from. These recipes not only taste great but also offer the added benefits of vitamins, minerals, and antioxidants from the fresh ingredients used.

Whether you're sipping these infused waters at home, at work, or on the go, you can feel good about making a healthy choice that keeps you hydrated and satisfies your taste buds. Plus, by sharing these recipes with friends and family, you can inspire others to enjoy the benefits of infused water as well.

So, keep exploring, keep experimenting, and most importantly, keep sipping! With this book as your guide, you'll never look at water the same way again. Cheers to your health and happiness, one delicious glass of infused water at a time!

My Words

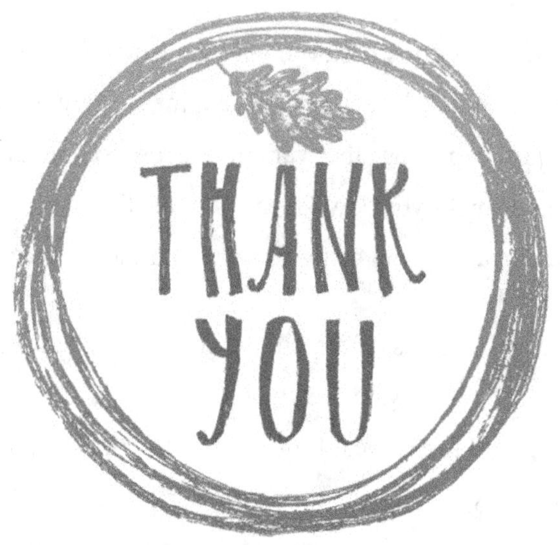

I cannot express enough how grateful I am for your decision to purchase my book. It is a humbling feeling to know that people are interested in learning from my experiences and the content that I have created. Being a writer has allowed me to share my knowledge and skills with others, and it is truly an honor to have you choose my book out of the multitude of books available on the market.

Your choice to invest in my book is incredibly special to me, and I am confident that the content you will find within its pages will prove to be valuable and insightful. It is my sincere hope that you will learn a great deal from the knowledge I have shared and that it will positively impact your life in some way.

After reading the book, I kindly request that you leave feedback, no matter how small. As a writer, I am always looking to improve and provide better content to my readers. Your feedback will be an invaluable source of information, and I will take it into consideration when creating future books. It is my goal to create content that my readers love and find helpful, and your input will play an important role in helping me achieve that.

Once again, I would like to express my gratitude for your support and for choosing my book. Your investment in my work means the world to me, and I am honored to have the opportunity to share my knowledge with you. Your feedback and support will be greatly appreciated and will help me to continue creating meaningful and valuable content for readers like you.

Kind regards,

Alex K. Aton